Respective authors own all copyrights not held by the publisher.

The information herein is offered for informational purposes solely and is universal as so. The presentation of the information is without contract or any type of guarantee assurance.

The trademarks that are used are without any consent, and the publication of the trademark is without permission or backing by the trademark owner. All trademarks and brands within this book are for clarifying purposes only and are the owned by the owners themselves, not affiliated with this document.

All health content found in this book is provided for general information only and should not be treated as a substitute for the medical advice of your own doctor or any other health care professional. If you have any concerns about your general health, you should contact your local health care provider.

Introduction

I want to thank you and congratulate you for purchasing this book:

'Menopause - A Complete Menopause Health and Wellness Guide.'

This book contains proven steps and strategies on how to understand and manage your pre-menopause/menopause and post-menopausal journey with knowledge and confidence.
This book covers a vast amount of information from pre-menopause all the way through to post-menopause including diet, lifestyle, natural alternatives to HRT and HRT. I cover how hormones affect your health, menopause and your well-being.

I also list vital foods to eat daily to achieve optimal health and to sail smoothly through the menopause with confidence. I list the foods and drinks which act as triggers for hot flushes and other unwanted symptoms. The book also educates you on symptoms and proven methods used to manage the many symptoms of menopause.

I have studied the menopause and women's health for over 20 years and have a mass of knowledge to share with you.

A little story about my pre-menopausal experience –

At the age of 39 years old, my life had changed overnight. I woke up a different person and felt like a broken vase that had been roughly glued back together with lots of pieces missing! I felt alienated from myself and very confused.

My GP and the few others I sought for advice were of little help. I suggested to my doctors that I may be in the pre-menopause yet they all gave the same response; "you are far too young to be in the menopause". It didn't help matters either when my blood tests came back inconclusive, early peri-menopause is difficult to detect via a blood test. I was offered anti-depressants and politely declined the offer.

I honestly felt like I was losing my sanity and as a divorced lone-parent of three sons, I felt rather alienated with my new chaotic, mind and body.

My symptoms were:

- foggy head, headaches, poor brain function, poor memory, confusion, anxiety and panic attacks, wanting to smile and laugh but feeling sad at the same time, insomnia and poor sleep patterns, dull slow thought processes, very painful and heavy periods, tender and painful breasts, increased appetite, sugar and carb cravings, weight gain, erratic mood swings, feelings of rage coming out of nowhere, acting 'out of character', irritable and completely exhausted. The constant erratic hormone fluctuations can lead to a hormonal depression which doctors may overlook to a diagnosis of psychological depression linked to a chemical imbalance in the brain.

How many ladies are given anti-depressants for depression when in fact the symptoms they are experiencing are the result of a hormonal imbalance as in the pre-menopause/menopause? Many ladies are not aware that the pre-menopause can begin in their 30s, I was one of those ladies. I did at one point agree with my doctor that I was suffering from depression only because I was depressed with how my symptoms were impacting my health and my daily life. I did not know how to think differently about my health at that time, my time was being swallowed up by working 70-hour weeks as well as raising my 3 sons and running a home as a divorced lone-parent. It seemed to be the norm to take anti-depressants just so I could cope better (but it made no difference) when all the time my body was being affected by the pre-menopause.

- I also suffered from bowel and bladder problems which were misdiagnosed as IBS and yet it should have been a diagnosis of prolapse of the bladder and rectum.

Self-educating is an absolute must. Knowledge is power after all, and at this stage of one's life it can be the difference between living a happy, normal life or a miserable and desperate existence. Living in chaos must be avoided and arming yourself with knowledge ready for when you pay a visit to your doctor will empower you, your health and your future health.

It must also be understood that a person may have any of the symptoms of the pre-menopause/menopause but may have another underlying health condition, so it is so highly important to see your doctor as soon as you feel unwell or just 'out of sorts'. I regularly see my healthcare professional every two months so she can keep a check on my health in general, as well as discussing my symptoms with me in depth and suggesting any relevant support available.

I find it disheartening that many women do feel confused, misguided and in a muddle moving through their menopause journey and this should not be allowed to continue. It is ultimately up to the individual to obtain the knowledge and know-how needed to help cope with the many symptoms and bodily changes with ease and confidence.

Working a job, juggling family commitments and finding the time to read for hours on end can be a challenge most of us tend to struggle with but I do hope you find the answers you were looking for in this book.

I have read many books on menopause, yet my muddled and foggy brain could not deal with the medical terms the doctors were using, and I found myself wanting a book that I could easily understand. Then came my idea of writing a book on the *"menopause journey"* in a simple fashion aimed at the ladies who are simply looking for an easier and informative read with no diversions.

I do sincerely hope this book helps you and thank-you!

Table of Contents

Chapter 9. The Positives of Post-Menopausal Living

1. Thinking positively

Chapter 1.

Pre-Menopause: The Hormonal Dance

There are 3 stages of the menopause:

- Pre-Menopause
- Menopause
- Post Menopause

What is the Pre-Menopause?

Another term for pre-menopause is "menopausal transition", which refers to the coming to the end of your reproductive life before you finally reach the menopause.

Pre-menopause begins several years before menopause. In your late 30s the egg supply within your ovaries begin to decline in number and in quality resulting in hormonal changes.

Every woman is unique but on average a woman will begin the pre-menopause from late 30s-40s onwards up to the mid/late 40s then moving into the menopause itself. There are cases where women have started their pre-menopause very early in life compared to the expected age groups, although this can be due to a medical condition. Women who have had a hysterectomy will automatically move into the menopause.

A percentage of women will experience a premature pre-menopause which can start in her early 30s, yet in some women the pre-menopause can begin later in her early 50s.

It is around this time that you may notice a change in your monthly periods. They may become erratic and irregular, shorter or longer, heavier and bearing more intense bouts of pain. It is common to experience spotting in-between periods, and you may even go several months without having one. Every woman experiences a different pattern.

What is happening to my reproductive organs now my periods are changing?

As the ovaries age, they release fewer of the hormones – **FSH** (follicle stimulating hormone) and **LH** (luteinizing hormone). FSH and LH can no longer perform their functions of regulating the hormones: oestrogen, progesterone and testosterone. The change of hormone levels and the decline of oestrogen can have a significant effect on your overall health and well-being.

The ovaries are now producing either too much oestrogen and/or progesterone or too little. The fluctuation of progesterone can result in heavier menstrual bleeding. Please note that a visit to your doctor is sensible to have your health checked just to make sure there are no other underlying health issues.

The shifting of these hormone levels can be an unsettling process and can affect one's sleep patterns.

What are the symptoms of pre-menopause?

Weight gain – the body responds to low levels of oestrogen by retaining more fat cells to increase oestrogen levels. The muscle mass decreases as we age. The depleting oestrogen levels can slow down the metabolism.

Reduced muscle mass is associated with the declining oestrogen levels. The negative effects are increased visceral fat, a reduction of bone mass density, muscle mass and strength.

Sore/tender/swollen breasts – due to hormonal fluctuations and increasing levels of progesterone.

Joint pain – caused by hormonal changes and imbalance. The decline of oestrogen negatively affects the joints and bones. A normal, healthy level of oestrogen protects our joints from inflammation.

Hot flushes/flashes – The hormonal fluctuations are one of the causes of hot flushes although other factors can also contribute.

Spotting – Bleeding in-between menstrual cycles.

Irregular and heavy bleeding – Fluctuating progesterone levels.

Mood swings – Oestrogen influences the production of serotonin which is a mood regulating transmitter. As oestrogen fluctuates brain functions are affected. There are other causes of mood swings too, but this will occur during the dance of the hormones.

Poor memory and cognitive function – There are many factors involved here, but as the hormones oestrogen and progesterone decline this can have a negative effect on brain performance. A reduced level of progesterone can lead to mood swings, brain fog and irritability. Insomnia is also linked to declining progesterone.

Anxiety and depression – hormone fluctuations, lack of quality sleep, life stresses can have a negative effect which can lead to low mood. Added to this are concerns about body image and infertility which can lead to emotional distress.

Low libido –

    a) Psychological – This is when a woman feels no emotional interest in sex.

    b) Physical – Due to the vaginal changes the woman loses interest in sex due to the lack of normal secretions which can lead to soreness.

Vaginal dryness – Oestrogen is responsible for keeping the vagina moist and plump but there is now a significant lowered level of this hormone resulting in vaginal dryness. The vaginal lips and vagina become less elastic and drier making intercourse uncomfortable. The vaginal glands also produce a lower level of mucus which can lead to vaginal dryness.

Insomnia – Due to sporadic changes in hormone levels, difficulty in sleeping may well occur. Hot flashes are caused by a surge of adrenalin which can wake the brain from sleep, often producing sweat and a change of temperature leading to a disrupted night's sleep.

Urinary incontinence – Oestrogen helps to keep our bladder and urethra healthy when at a normal level. As this hormone starts to deplete, our organs do not work as efficiently as they should. The lack of oestrogen can contribute to the pelvic floor muscles weakening leading to urinary incontinence. There are three types of incontinence;

Stress Incontinence – is the most common of all bladder disorders amongst menopausal and post-menopausal women. Weakened muscles cannot efficiently hold the urine when we cough, laugh, exercise, lift something heavy or sneeze, resulting in leakage. This can also occur as result of pregnancy and childbirth too.

Urge incontinence – is when the bladder muscles contract abnormally or lose the ability to naturally relax, which can lead to a constant feeling or urge that you want to urinate even when the bladder is empty. You may also experience 'leakage of urine' or loss of control. This is called an 'overactive bladder'.

Overflow incontinence – is when the bladder does not empty completely, resulting in a constant 'dribbling' of urine loss. This can be caused when there is an underactivity of the bladder muscle.

Prolapse - Increased risk of the bladder, rectum and uterus prolapsing is very common in women going through the menopause (even earlier) especially if they have had vaginal births and are carrying excess body fat.
It is so important at this stage of one's life to lose any excess weight and achieve your ideal body weight. Obesity and carrying excess fat will only increase the risk of developing a prolapse. It would be very beneficial to start activities such as Pilates and

Yoga to help to keep the pelvic floor muscles tight and strong. Kegel exercises are very helpful too in strengthening the pelvic floor muscles.

Interstitial Cystitis – this is a chronic neuroinflammatory disorder which affects the bladder. It involves the bladder nerves, urinary tract and the immune system.
If it is left untreated IC can lead to scarring, an inability to hold urine in the bladder and rigidity of the bladder walls.
The symptoms of IC can be mistaken for other conditions such as UTI's (urinary tract infections), STD's (sexually transmitted diseases), endometriosis, kidney stones, urge incontinence and bladder cancer.

The symptoms of IC are:
- pelvic and bladder pain
- unable to hold much urine
- urinary urgency and frequency
- ulcers (Hunner's ulcers – rare)

Dry eyes – This is a common complaint of one of the symptoms of menopause and is yet not totally understood why this occurs. One major factor could be, due to hormone levels becoming erratic and unbalanced, the composition of tears is therefore affected. Dry eyes can become irritated with a gritty feeling on blinking. Tear fluid doesn't seem to protect the eyes enough against environmental factors, such a weather and temperature.

To help relieve dry eyes, it is important to drink plenty of water to stay hydrated as one of the first places your body will take fluid from is the eyes.

Chapter 2.

How do I know if I am in the Menopause?

The menopause begins when periods have completely ceased (usually) for 12 months at least. The eggs stop being released by the ovaries and hormone levels begin to decline. Through the lack of oestrogen (which normally keeps the vagina moist and plump) women experience vaginal dryness, although this can often happen in the peri-menopause too. Another common symptom of being in the menopause is a strong loss of libido, painful intercourse and low mood which can lead to depression. The symptoms of menopause are very like the ones listed in the pre-menopause chapter.

How will I know I am in Post-Menopause?

There are no actual symptoms to know that you are out of the menopause and into the post-menopause phase. If the menstrual cycles have been stopped for a whole 12 months, then this is when the menopause shifts towards post-menopause.

During post-menopause, your hormone levels will not usually fluctuate to the same extent as they did during the lead-up to menopause, which means that many women do find symptom relief from entering the postmenopausal phase. It is a very different experience for each individual woman.

Many women report their energy levels increase and they feel much more 'normal'. There are several factors at play here, but as the oestrogen and progesterone levels are now low, there are increased health risks for certain health conditions, such as heart disease and osteoporosis. These risks can be managed by adopting a healthy lifestyle and a healthy diet.

What are the symptoms of Post-Menopause?

As hormone levels are (not for every woman) now in a permanently lowered state, there are many symptoms which can be experienced and these symptoms can also be experienced during pre-menopause. There are women who will experience hormone fluctuations for many years throughout the post-menopause phase. These symptoms include, stress, insomnia, weight gain and hot flushes.

Once again, the pre-menopause/menopause/post-menopause experience is different for every woman based on how her body uniquely adapts to the ageing process.

The following symptoms are commonly reported as symptoms of Post-Menopause:

Weight gain - can be caused by the body's response to the lowering oestrogen levels, the reaction is to retain more fat cells to enable the oestrogen levels to increase.

Insomnia – the hormonal changes have a direct negative effect on the ability to naturally fall asleep along with disrupted sleep patterns.

Vaginal dryness – the lack of oestrogen can cause the vaginal lips and vagina to become less elastic. This will result in painful intercourse and soreness. A lower level of mucous production can also cause vaginal dryness.

Vaginal bleeding – once a woman has ceased to menstruate for at least 12 months and begins to experience vaginal bleeding, it may be classed as abnormal. It can be a common problem and can be caused by something minor such as inflammation or a thickened lining of the womb. It is very important to have this checked by your GP to rule out any underlying issues.

Urinary incontinence – oestrogen works to maintain a healthy bladder and urethra, which is the passage that urine passes through. Lowered hormone levels can result in bladder control problems. A normal level of oestrogen will help to keep the pelvic muscles strong and healthy, although now the oestrogen hormone is depleted this can result in weakened pelvic muscles which will in turn affect bladder control.

Most postmenopausal women will find that these symptoms diminish as their hormone levels stabilize. A percentage of women report the continuation of various symptoms that can last up to 10 years or so after menopause. Hot flushes, joint pain, mood swings, low libido and fatigue may continue until a woman is in her late 60s.

The Importance of Health and Nutrition

Nutrition and lifestyle are major factors of minimizing health-related illnesses and disease. This applies to every stage of a woman's life, but holds vastly more importance now as the body is undergoing so many natural changes. Regular exercise will always work in your favor; be kind to your body and it shall reward you.

A woman going through the menopause and beyond will need to adjust her diet according to the body's specific needs. To help prevent osteoporosis it is advised to increase calcium intake and vitamin D daily. As we age our blood vessels become less elastic which can increase our risks of developing high blood pressure. To help reduce these risks we need to reduce the salt intake and increase our healthy fats, such as omega 3, to support heart health.

Now is the perfect time to begin a major overhaul of every area of your life. See it as the ultimate mass detox to eliminate any unnecessary bad habits in your lifestyle choices. The mindset can be a destructive tool or a very powerful one, so use it wisely. The less stress we have, the smaller the impact on our bodies. This can be a very wonderful and very liberating stage of our life if we choose it to be. We are full of unique experiences, wisdom and beauty. Ageing can be beautiful if we learn to embrace it and respect it, not fight it.

We can take plenty of measures to become, slimmer, fitter, healthier, more youthful, sexier, more confident, and much more successful in every way we choose. This is a choice designed by you only for you. I see the menopause as a gift, a chance to reinvent my whole self, my lifestyle and to be a richer person in every way possible.

How often do I need to see my GP/Doctor during my Post-menopause?

The Post-menopause is with you for the rest of your life and therefore having regular health checks are very important. Preventative screening tests are necessary and tests such as pelvic exams, breast exams, mammograms and cervical smears are all required to be done regularly. Self-help, such as checking your breasts for lumps, is important too. Your health and medical history will determine how often your GP and hospital visits are required. Talk to your doctor to determine how often you should be seen.

Chapter 3.

The Endocrine System

All the body's organs are relying heavily on the hormones being delivered to them to perform their necessary function to keep everything working in sync. Just one hormonal imbalance can have a very negative effect on one's overall health and the whole hormonal balance system can be placed under stress.

The hormonal system is called 'The Endocrine System' and this is the foundation of glands and hormones. The Endocrine System influences almost every cell in the human body, every organ and the general functioning of the human body. It also holds a significant role in the regulation of growth and development, mood, tissue function, sexual function, metabolism and the reproductive system.

The endocrine glands secrete their hormones directly into the blood and are delivered to the organs where needed.
The major glands of a woman's endocrine system include:

- pituitary gland
- hypothalamus
- pineal gland
- pancreas
- ovaries
- thyroid gland
- parathyroid gland

- adrenal glands

The physical well-being of a woman during her menopausal years is linked strongly to how well her Endocrine System is functioning. To understand its importance during menopause will be useful, even if basic information is all that can be gathered.

- **The Pituitary Gland** is normally around the size of a pea and is located deep in the skull, behind the bridge of the nose. It is attached to the base of the skull by a thin stalk. This gland is referred to as the 'master gland' as it controls several other hormone glands in the body such as the thyroid, adrenals and ovaries.

- **Hypothalamus** is located immediately above the pituitary gland and controls the pituitary gland by sending it messages in the form of hormones. The hypothalamus influences the healthy functioning of emotional behavior, memory, sleep and wake patterns, temperature regulation, food ingestion and water intake.

- **The Pineal Gland** is located deep in the brain in the epithalamus which is where the two halves of the brain join. Its role is to secrete the hormone called melatonin which is responsible for the regulating of sleep patterns also known as circadian rhythms. The pineal gland also plays a role in the regulation of female hormones linked to fertility and the menstrual cycle.

- **The Pancreas** is located in the abdomen. The pancreas operates two main functions: an endocrine function which regulates sugar and an exocrine function which aids in digestion. The pancreas also helps to convert food into energy for the body's cells.
- **The Ovaries** are a part of the reproductive system and are located at the ends of the fallopian tubes. They produce the sex hormones oestrogen and progesterone. Ovulation takes place in the ovaries which occurs normally once a month known as the menstrual cycle.
- **The Thyroid Gland** is a small, bow-tie shaped organ located in the front of the neck above the collarbone. The main role of the thyroid gland is to produce the thyroid hormones – T3 (tr-iodothyronine) and T4 (thyroxine) which regulates the metabolism. If the thyroid gland is not functioning as it should, this can have a significant effect on one's energy level and mood.

1. **Hyperthyroidism** can cause weight loss, disrupted sleep patterns, anxiety, irritability and restlessness.
2. **Hypothyroidism** is another thyroid disorder causing weight gain, depression and extreme fatigue.

- **The Pararthyroid Glands** are small glands located in the neck behind the thyroid gland. They control the calcium levels in the bones, blood and entire body. Calcium is one of the most important elements and is used by the body to control many of its systems. Calcium is used by our body to:
- to provide the electrical energy for the nervous system
- to provide the electrical energy for the muscular system

- to provide strength to the skeletal system

- **The Adrenal Glands** are located on the top of each kidney. Each adrenal gland is made up of two parts which are called: the adrenal cortex (the outer part) and the inner adrenal medulla. The adrenal glands secrete different hormones and are known as 'chemical messengers'. The hormones travel into the bloodstream and are delivered to various body tissues to perform a necessary function. The main hormones produced by the adrenal glands are, aldosterone and cortisol. Aldosterone helps to regulate the body's salt and water levels which then regulates the blood pressure. Cortisol supports and regulates the stress response as well as supporting the metabolism. Cortisol stimulates glucose production by mobilizing amino acids and fatty free acids. Cortisol also has powerful anti-inflammatory effects on the body.

Adrenal Fatigue can be overlooked by most doctors resulting in a misdiagnosis of this condition. They often prescribe anti-depressants or Hormone Replacement Therapy as the symptoms of adrenal fatigue can be like symptoms of the menopause.

The effects of the menopause, everyday general life stressors, an unbalanced diet, poor sleep patterns and little exercise can all have a negative effect on the adrenal glands. When there is a hormone imbalance this can also put extra stress on other glands and chaos begins. Such compounded stress over time will eventually lead to adrenal fatigue. The symptoms include:

- poor quality sleep
- low mood, anxiety and depression
- hot flushes
- headaches
- painful joints
- digestive issues
- itchy skin
- Feelings of nausea – the list goes on.

Can you see how this disorder can be so easily misdiagnosed? They are all quite like the symptoms of the menopause.

Self-education is paramount especially at this stage of one's life.

As you can see if these other very important glands are not functioning as they should then most of the resulting symptoms could be mistaken as those of the menopause and post menopause. The last thing that is needed at this stage of one's life is to suffer from more hormone/gland issues. A visit to an endocrinologist would be very wise at this stage of one's life to have every hormone level checked within the endocrine system.

Chapter 4.

A Brief Overview on Female Hormones

Oestrogen is a hormone produced mainly in the ovaries. It is also produced by the adrenal gland and the fat cells. Oestrogen boosts the synthesis and function of neurotransmitters in the brain which influence libido, mood, memory, sleep and cognitive functioning such as attention span and learning.

The roles of Oestrogen are responsible for the growth and development of female secondary sexual characteristics such as armpit and pubic hair, breasts, wider hips, endometrium and the functioning of the menstrual cycle and reproductive system.

Oestrogen also:

- increases HDL – the good cholesterol
- protects our bones and joint health.
- protects against heart disease. Dilates the blood vessels and prevents harmful plaques from building up in the vessel walls.
- is important in efficiently regulating the fluid levels in the body.
- plays an important role in the health and elasticity of the vagina
- is related to hair growth and health
- supports muscle function, helps to keep the pelvic floor muscles strong
- preserves the elasticity and moisture content of the skin

Oestrogen normally helps to keep our ligaments and muscles strong but once the pre-menopause begins we are more at risk of prolapses as the oestrogen declines. Obesity can increase the possibility of being diagnosed with a prolapse so the earlier we adopt positive lifestyle changes to lose excess weight and increase our fitness the lesser the risk.

Progesterone is a hormone produced mainly by the corpus luteum which is inside the ovary. The corpus luteum is the body which is left over after a follicle has released an egg. Progesterone is responsible for the thickening of the lining of the womb in preparation for implantation of a fertilized egg. If the egg is not fertilized then the progesterone production stops, once the progesterone levels drop the uterus lining stops thickening and menstruation begins. Progesterone is also produced in the adrenal glands and in the placenta during pregnancy.

Progesterone binds to certain receptors in the brain to induce a sedating and calming effect. It can also help to improve sleep and can protect against seizures.

Testosterone is a male hormone but is also produced in Women in small amounts in the ovaries and adrenal glands. Testosterone helps to regulate sex drive (libido), energy and mental well-being. It helps to strengthen ligaments, the formation of muscle and bone, supports brain function and an overall feeling of well-being. Testosterone contributes to the prevention of cardiovascular disease in both sexes.

Collagen is the most abundant protein in the body. It plays a major role in the formation of bones, ligaments, tendons, muscles and skin. It is also responsible for providing structure to the skin and helping blood to clot. Collagen is found in many other bodily structures including, blood vessels, corneas and teeth. It is similar in description as a form of human "glue" which holds of these structures together. Collagen is found throughout the entire body and there are at least 16 types of collagen. As the body ages, it produces it produces less collagen and of a lower quality.

Collagen is a fibrous protein and it provides structural support for tissues and cells. The benefits of collagen are as follows:

- maintains the strength and elasticity of the skin
- strengthens nails and hair/hair growth
- bone strength and the prevention of osteoporosis
- promotes healthy eye vision
- protects the walls of blood vessels
- prevents cancer metastasis
- helps to fight body fats

From the age of 25 collagen begins to deplete and fine lines and wrinkles are noticeable.

Chapter 5.

Diet and Nutrition – Always shop for organic and NON-GMO foods

Is soy good for you or bad for you?

The processed or GMO soy is bad for your health. Alarmingly, 90% of soy today is genetically modified (GMO). Genetically modified food products kill off the good gut bacteria and are linked to many health conditions, they can also damage the digestive system. The bad soy includes soy protein, soy milk and any other soy product out there unless it a soy lecithin (organic non-gmo) which is safe to consume. Try drinking goat milk or coconut milk which has many health benefits. The good soy to consume is an organic, fermented soy which means there are no chemicals, pesticides or fertilizers used. When a food is fermented it increases its probiotic value. The body is full of good and bad bacteria, probiotics are live "good" bacteria helping to maintain optimum gut health.

A soy called "natto" is consumed heavily by the people who live in Okinawa, Japan and live to be 100 years old and older. Natto is one of the healthiest fermented foods and is loaded with probiotics, high in a vitamin called vitamin K2 and is non-GMO. Vitamin K2 helps to build strong bones, supports brain health and promotes natural healing within the body. Fermented soy is awesome for one's health. Adding the supplement K2 to your daily diet is very wise, do a search online and look for MK-7. Always see your doctor before adding supplements to your diet.

Cheese is high in a protein called proline which is an amino acid. This amino acid is needed for production of cartilage and collagen. Proline also helps to keep the muscles and joints flexible and aids in the prevention of skin ageing.

Lysine is another amino acid that is needed by the body to produce collagen. Lentils are an excellent source of Lysine. As an approximate guide, adults are recommended to eat 12mg of lysine per 1kg of the body weight daily. Lentils are one of the best vegan food sources rich in lysine.

Beans contain anti-ageing properties and are packed with antioxidants. Antioxidants are man-made or natural substances that may prevent or delay some forms of cell damage.

FACT: Just a half cup of dried red kidney or pinto beans contains some of the highest amounts of anti-oxidants in any food.

Hyaluronic acid is a carbohydrate which is found in the body's tissues. As we age, the natural HA levels decrease so it is essential to eat foods which are going to help your body to produce more. HA builds collagen, supports skin cell renewal and helps in the healing of wounds.

The best foods containing hyaluronic acid are:

- Bone Broth is very rich in hyaluronic acid. The broth comes from beef, chicken and other meats. Slow cooking the bones, skin, cartilage and ligaments for up to 24 hours is best. Once fully cooked, important nutrients are released which include hyaluronic acid, magnesium, calcium and potassium.

- Non-GMO soy foods such as natto, tofu, tempeh, miso, soy milk, soy sauce, soy pasta and soy yoghurt contain properties which raise oestrogen levels, in turn this will raise the hyaluronic acid levels. The isoflavones in these foods enable this effect.
- Red Wine drunk in moderation is an excellent source of hyaluronic acid. The wine contains the skin of red grapes which is a vital source of phytoestrogen.
- Root Vegetables contain the highest amount (compared to other vegetables) of hyaluronic acid. Theses consist of sweet potatoes, potatoes, carrots, and lotus roots. There are many others too. There is a theory which states that high levels of magnesium found in root vegetables enables the body to process an even higher amount of hyaluronic acid.

Dark green vegetables are an excellent source of food for collagen production. Spinach, cabbage and kale eaten daily will also give the body an antioxidant called lutein. Lutein is also beneficial for eye health. It is recommended to consume 10 mg of lutein rich foods daily to achieve the benefits. This would equate to approximately 4oz spinach or 2oz kale.

There has been recent research suggesting that this will also boost skin hydration and elasticity keeping the skin less prone to premature ageing. These dark leafy vegetables (including collards and asparagus) eaten daily can help the body to manufacture its collagen and enable it to utilize the protein effectively. This also means stronger and healthier cells throughout.

Vegetables and red fruits have many health benefits but are also excellent in helping the body to top up on its collagen stores. These foods contain lycopenes which are a form of antioxidant and has cancer-preventing properties. The list of health benefits is vast if eaten daily. Red tomatoes are very rich in lycopene. The antioxidant property of lycopene increases collagen production. Red, yellow and orange foods contain specific antioxidants that build up under the skin helping to prevent against UV damage. These foods eaten daily will give other amazing health benefits too.

One of the biggest factors which contributes to skin ageing is it being attacked by free radicals. Environment plays a big role in exposing ourselves to free radicals such as, pollution, toxic metals, alcohol, cigarette smoke, radiation, industrial chemicals and medications. Cellular metabolism also exposes us to free radicals.

Eating a diet rich in antioxidants can help to neutralize these free radicals before they can cause damage to the body.

Prunes contain an abundance of antioxidants compared to other fruits, blueberries come in at second place.

Foods rich in Omega acids are, tuna, salmon and mackerel. Other foods high in omega 3 are, flaxseed oil, fish oil, chia seeds, eggs, soybeans and spinach. They contribute to an ideal environment for collagen production. Omega acids are also found in various nuts such as, almonds, brazil nuts, cashews, and pecan.

Coconut Oil is classed as a true "superfood." The benefits include weight loss, skin health, prevents heart disease, high blood pressure, reduces inflammation and arthritis but the list goes on and on. Coconut oil contains a large amount of medium chain triglycerides and can have therapeutic effects on several brain disorders. Coconut oil can help the body to burn more fat. Always buy the cold pressed, virgin, organic coconut oil as this is the purest form.

Active Manuka Honey has been recommended for the relief of menopause symptoms. The Maori people of New Zealand have been using it for skin care for centuries. Manuka honey (when used topically) can restore and rejuvenate the skin supporting in the formation of collagen production. A daily dose of Manuka can help to fight off – dry skin, digestive issues and bloating. Many use it for hair health and to combat acne and skin blemishes. It is said to have a healing effect in many ways.

Dark Chocolate can be very beneficial to health especially if it contains a minimum 70-85% cocoa content. Just 100g of dark chocolate will provide your body with fibre, iron, magnesium, copper, manganese, potassium, phosphorous, zinc and selenium. A very tasty way to treat your body to essential minerals.

Green Tea is a great substitute for replacing tea and coffee as it is full of anti-oxidants and can increase the metabolism which can help weight-loss. It does contain caffeine but not as much as tea or coffee. Herbal teas are a great alternative too.

*Try to avoid snacking on sugary, high processed foods as these will cause a sharp increase in your blood glucose levels which will crash just as fast leaving you with little energy and lethargy. Eating fresh fruit, seeds and nuts are a great alternative and your body and mind will thank you.

*Cut out (or reduce) drinks and foods that will worsen the hot flushes such as; coffee, alcohol, spicy foods. This is important especially at night when these foods could trigger or make the hot flushes more intense.

We are taught to expect gain weight going through the pre-menopause, menopause and thereafter. As our bodies mature we need fewer calories so eating fewer calories makes sense to keep control of this. Cut back on saturated fats, sugar and processed foods too. Start to move more and often.

Foods to achieve optimal health

Eat plenty of complex carbs such as; wholegrains, brown rice, whole meal bread, and whole meal pasta. These will help to control blood sugars for longer and keep you fuller to avoid cravings. The fibre is also very beneficial to your gut health and can help to prevent diverticulitis and other disorders of the bowel.

Dry skin, spots and acne can be a problem too as the hormones decline so eating a diet rich in vitamin e, zinc and calcium is a must. Foods rich in these are legumes, nuts and seeds. Pumpkin and sunflower seeds are rich in vitamin e and zinc. Almonds are rich in healthy fats, fibre, protein, magnesium and vitamin e.

The benefits of almonds include – reduced blood sugar levels, reduced cholesterol and reduced blood pressure. They can also help to crush cravings and aid in weight loss. The oils and nutrients in the nuts and seeds may help to prevent dry skin and tame those hormone fluctuations. Other essential fatty acids for skin health are omega 3s found in salmon and oily fish. These smart fatty acids help strengthen the skin's natural oil barrier maintaining skin hydration. Sardines, soy, safflower oil and flax are rich in omega 3s too.

Depression and irritability - Eating foods rich in the amino acid tryptophan are important as it acts as a sort of mood regulator and has a calming effect. Eating foods rich in tryptophan can also help to maintain a healthy hormone balance. Tryptophan can also help to induce sleep, fights anxiety and can even help in burning more body fat. Foods rich in tryptophan are – nuts, seeds, tofu, cheese, cottage cheese, red meat, chicken, turkey, fish, oats, beans, lentils and eggs.

Eating breakfast too is important to avoid irritability and sugar crashes. Aim to not miss a meal throughout the day. I eat every 4 hours and no food after 7pm (only water), it really does work.

Bone Health

Women can lose up to 20% of their bone density 5 to 7 years after the menopause. Oestrogen helps to protect bone strength, As the oestrogen declines during menopause it is ever so important to eat foods rich in calcium, magnesium, vitamins d and k such as – green leafy vegetables, nuts, seeds, dried fruit, salmon, tinned fish with bones and dairy products like milk, yoghurt and cheese. Aim to drink the low fat or no fat milk as there is still the same calcium amount as in full fat milk. Vitamin d rich foods are – oily fish, eggs, foods fortified with vitamin d such as – cereals, soy milk and orange juice.

Eat foods high in boron such as – apples, pears, grapes, dates, raisins, legumes and nuts are all good sources of boron. Boron assists in absorbing calcium and aids in increasing bone mass. Exercise also helps the body absorb calcium.

Vitamin D

Vitamin d is naturally produced by the skin when it is exposed to sunlight and is required by the body to process calcium and phosphorous absorption. It is needed for the health of bones, muscles and teeth. Vitamin d plays an important role in the prevention of brittle bone disease and fracture. It is said that Vitamin d will also give a protective effect against diseases such as cancer and conditions such as multiple sclerosis and diabetes. Important to note that most of our vitamin d will come from sunshine and is naturally found in very few foods. This vitamin is added to certain foods by the manufacturer. Fatty fish such as tuna, mackerel and salmon are among the best sources. Small amounts of vitamin d are found in cheese, beef liver and egg yolks.

It is wise to go and see your doctor to have your vitamin d levels checked through a blood test. I did this and my levels were too low resulting in a vitamin deficiency, I was prescribed a high dose of vitamin d to take daily. I did feel much better after 6 weeks of taking them. Taking a daily walk to soak up the natural light and sunshine is important too.

Are phytoestrogens good or bad for our health?

Phytoestrogens are compounds that are naturally found in plants and are plant-based oestrogens. They are rather mysterious to understand. Their effects are somewhat controversial and research findings is found to be conflicted. What makes them tricky to understand is their ability to mimic oestrogen and in also acting as an oestrogen antagonist (behaving in the opposite way of biological oestrogen).

When consumed, phytoestrogens attach themselves to oestrogen receptors but as they are not actually needed for the human diet they are not considered as actual nutrients.

Many health benefits are linked to a diet consisting of phytoestrogens including a lowered risk of osteoporosis and menopausal symptoms, but many phytoestrogens are also considered to be endocrine disruptors. This means that they have the potential to cause negative health effects. It still is not proven if phytoestrogens are beneficial or harmful to health.

Many factors would be needed to be considered such as health status, age and the absence or presence of specific gut microflora. The answer is still likely to be complex and there needs to be more research undertaken to reassure the consumer of it's true health effects. Phytoestrogens are being marketed as natural alternative to oestrogen replacement therapy and are present in many dietary supplements.

Foods rich in phytoestrogens are:

NON-GMO organic soy products, tempeh, flaxseeds, oats, barley, lentils, sesame seeds, yams, alfalfa, apples, carrots, jasmine oil, pomegranates, wheatgerm, coffee, hops, bourbon, beer, red clover and clary sage oil.

Phytoestrogens are compounds that are naturally found in plants and are plant-based oestrogens. They are rather mysterious to understand. Their effects are somewhat controversial and research findings is found to be conflicted. What makes them tricky to understand is their ability to mimic

When consumed, phytoestrogens attach themselves to oestrogen receptors but as they are not actually needed for the human diet they are not considered as actual nutrients.

There is an area of confusion regarding the positive and negative consumption of phytoestrogens.

Here are a few positives:

- Phytoestrogens have a positive effect on certain types of cancers such as, hormonal cancers, breast cancer and ovarian cancer.
- They are good for your heart health and help to treat atherosclerosis.
- They help to improve health during menopause by counteracting the hormonal imbalances.
- Phytoestrogens contain genistein which helps to fight obesity.
- Phytoestrogens in alcoholic beverages are said to help increase libido.

Here are a few negatives:

- A diet high in phytoestrogens can adversely affect fertility and polycystic ovarian syndrome.
- Eating low consumption of phytoestrogens can negatively affect hormone health and may stimulate breast cancer growth.
- An increased risk of dementia and cognitive decline.

Doctors do make mistakes (they are only human) and may misdiagnose their patients from time to time. I am one of those patients and so was my deceased Mother. My Mother was diagnosed of acidity at the age of 45 and prescribed Gaviscon to treat it, at the age of 46 she died of cancer of the stomach and esophagus.

This very painful experience taught me at the age of 17 (I am now 50) to self-educate constantly and to do whatever it takes to understand and get to know my mind and body as well as I possibly can. Only *we* know how *we* live day by day, only *we* know the risks we take with our lives and health. That said, even the healthiest of people can become ill but we must still do all we can to ensure we are doing everything possible to stay in good health.

The doctor can only do so much with the information we give them. We of course need our doctors but we can do our absolute best to avoid illness and disease by choosing our food and lifestyle choices wisely. You are your very best friend but you can also be your worst enemy.

Allergies

I have spent my last 40 years being crippled daily by allergies and not one doctor has ever treated the cause but only treated the symptoms with medication that made it all the worse and gave me new health problems. I now follow an anti-inflammatory diet which has eliminated my allergens by 90%. I researched and tried the elimination diet, I lived by the 'sword of truth' (my pen and pad) to note every reaction after eating and drinking foods and fluids, the ingesting of minerals, vitamins, medications and supplements as I am allergic to most of everything sold in the supermarkets and pharmacies.

The foods we eat are vital to our health, how frustrating and overwhelming it is to eat the healthiest foods only to become suddenly unwell. Food allergies are often overlooked and misdiagnosed. A food intolerance can be devastating to our health and well-being. A histamine is a chemical that is made in the immune system, aiding in efficient digestion and the central nervous system. It acts as a neurotransmitter communicating and relaying messages via the body to the brain. It is also found in the stomach acid which will help to break the food down in the stomach.

The histamine's primary role is to eliminate something which is causing an abnormal or harmful reaction in the the body. This could be from an allergic reaction to ingested food, drink, various pollens, dust, animal fur and saliva, insect bites, topical irritants, vitamin/mineral/health supplements and medication. Histamine is released when the body is fighting an infection or a virus, the blood flow is increased to the area under attack.

Histamine Intolerance

Histamine intolerance is when a histamine has entered the body via certain foods, a reaction is caused as the food moves through the digestion process. Normally, a digestive enzyme found in the gut called diamine oxidase will break down the histamine caused by certain foods but if there isn't enough of this enzyme then this will lead to a build-up of histamine. This then produces many uncomfortable symptoms such as tummy pain, diarrhea, nausea, joint pain, headaches, hives, itching, sneezing, asthma, eczema and rashes.

The histamine intolerance can be extreme and debilitating for many people and the factors to be considered are, genetics, allergies, diet, medications, environment, nutritional deficiencies, intestinal damage and UV exposure.

A food allergy test will not be of use for this condition. A blood test to check the levels of the enzyme diamine oxidase will determine if this is condition is present. If you are on a low-histamine diet at the time of the testing then the results are likely to be inaccurate.

The Histamine and Oestrogen Link

This condition is very important as it is yet another one that is often misdiagnosed and once in the pre-menopause/menopause it can bring more discomfort and general poor health.

As we move through the dance of the hormones we are encountering many symptoms we really do not want. Pain and inflammation in the body can be caused by a low progesterone to oestrogen ratio which is associated with increased levels of molecules which will cause inflammation.

These molecules are called Kinins and the oestrogen increases the kinin levels yet progesterone can decrease them. Kinins promote the release of histamines. Too much histamine in the body are linked to bowel diseases, asthma, psoriatic arthritis and rheumatoid arthritis. These high levels of kinins are linked to all conditions of allergic inflammation.

You can see why there is so much more to understanding what can be happening inside of your body. There is a strong link between high histamine levels and hormonal imbalances. There is also a strong link between high histamine levels and hot flushes. Please do read more on histamine intolerance and how they affect your hormones. Learn to avoid foods which are high in histamines and eat the foods which are low in histamines which will help to reduce pain and inflammation.

Chapter 6.
Physical Activities

Walking has a very positive impact on health overall.
The benefits of walking are:
- calorie burning, increasing the body's metabolic rate, even when resting.
- stress control and the regulating of hormones
- reduction of lethargy and fatigue

Research has proven that walking has a positive effect on reducing menopausal symptoms and depression. The benefits were also said to have an enhancing effect on one's physical self-esteem.

Walking helps to build and tone muscle which then will lead to more fat loss as the more muscle we have the faster we burn off fat. Taking regular daily walks will also fight against diseases such as, heart disease, stroke and diabetes. Fast paced walking is not necessarily needed as slow-paced walking may burn calories faster as the body is forced to carry its weight at a slower pace which forces more exertion.

Evidence suggests that being physically active on a regular basis can reduce the risk of three types of cancer – bowel cancer, womb cancer and breast cancer after the menopause.

Cardio activity

Cardio activity is any activity which increases your heart rate to approximately 50-75% of your maximum heart rate. Always consult a professional before undertaking any forms of moderate to intense activity.

A stronger heart and circulatory system will deliver more oxygen and nutrients to the body which will have a very positive impact overall.

Examples are: Walking, Running, tennis, dancing, jogging, biking, swimming and all activities which increase the heart-rate.

Cardio also improves brain function and fights against depression and anxiety. More benefits are improved sleep patterns and increased bone density which during menopause is very much needed.

Strength training

Strength training is very important for ladies going through menopause as due to the lack of oestrogen our bones are no longer protected. The risk of Osteoporosis is now increased and is referred to as the "silent disease" as there are no symptoms.

The benefits of strength training are, muscle growth and strength, increasing and strengthening new bone growth, burning of body fat and the speeding up your metabolism.

Yoga and meditation

Women going through the menopause are greatly supported by the benefits of yoga.

The benefits of yoga are:

- reduced stress, anxiety and depression
- physical pain and general discomfort is significantly reduced

- a sense of inner peace and calmness
- lowered blood pressure and less hot flush attacks

Yoga is also a natural remedy which is very beneficial to health. Vedic meditation can be comforting whilst going through the menopause as it can deal with many of the menopause symptoms which can mean the menopause can be moved through without HRT. Learn how to meditate the Vedic way.

Pilates

Pilates just like yoga is essential for the mind, body and overall health as the stretching actions of Pilates can help strengthen the bones and muscles. The benefits are:

- enabling you to have an open mind and to feel more positive, focused and motivated towards moving through the menopause with a healthy and invigorated mindset.
- improves blood circulation and eases muscle fatigue
- strengthens and tightens the pelvic floor muscles in helping to prevent prolapses of the uterus, bladder and rectum.
- the mind is quietened and this helps to soothe the nervous system.
- improves core strength and posture
- improved flexibility
- reduced body fat
- protecting the spine's natural alignment resulting in fewer back problems

Chapter 7.

Hormone Replacement Therapy for Menopause

HRT – as it is widely known is a treatment used to relieve the menopausal symptoms. It is designed to replace the depleting hormones throughout the pre-menopausal/menopausal transition.

The Benefits of HRT

HRT can relieve menopausal symptoms such as hot flushes, night sweats, mood swings, vaginal dryness, bladder symptoms and it can improve the libido. HRT can also help to strengthen and protect bones to reducing the risk of osteoporosis which is very common as women move through the ageing process. Taking HRT is said to also reduce the risks of heart attacks and from stroke. Women have reported that HRT has improved their sleep, mood and overall well-being leading to a better quality of life. They also report that the foggy brain feeling has lifted helping them to think more clearly, their energy levels have increased too.

We covered that a lack of oestrogen can negatively affect the skin and hair, HRT will increase the oestrogen levels resulting in thicker hair and healthier skin.

Many women are reluctant to start HRT due to the reports stating that they will be at an increased risk of certain cancers. Recent evidence has been published by the National Institute for Health and Care Excellence's (NICE), their new guidelines state that the risks of HRT are relatively small and the risks are normally outweighed by the benefits.

The Risks Associated with HRT

According to NICE the combined HRT (oestrogen and progesterone) is associated with a small elevated risk of breast cancer. Various studies have stated that for every 1,000 women using the combined HRT, five extra cases of breast cancer will be reported. To make it a little clearer, based on a normal risk of 22 cases of breast cancer per 1,000 menopausal women, this has increased to 27 cases on average. This is according to NICE.

The risk of breast cancer will decrease once the HRT treatment is stopped, it is suggested that the elevated risk associated with taking HRT will return to normal after 5 years. Oestrogen HRT taken without progesterone has proven to have little or no change in the increased risk of breast cancer.

As there is the associated link between HRT and breast cancer, it is very important to attend regular breast cancer screening appointments.

Ovarian Cancer:

The studies performed on the link between HRT and ovarian cancer are somewhat conflicted in their result findings. It is suggested that if there is a link between HRT and ovarian cancer then it is very small.

A recent study stated that for every 1,000 women taking HRT over a 5-year period, there will be one extra case of ovarian cancer. Once again, once HRT is stopped then this risk will be decreased.

Womb Cancer:
HRT which is oestrogen-only can increase the risk of cancer of the womb, also called endometrial cancer. This type of HRT is only used in women who have had their womb removed which is called a hysterectomy.

This risk is largely reduced if the HRT is taken in the combined form – progesterone and oestrogen continuously without a break. Doctors will ensure that women who do have a womb and are taking HRT will be prescribed the combined HRT to avoid the risk of womb cancer.

Blood Clots
If a blood clot becomes lodged in a blood vessel, this can be serious as it can block the blood flow. According to NICE:

- taking HRT orally in tablet form can increase the risk of blood clots

- taking HRT via a patch or gel form has no increased risk of developing a blood clot

- it is suggested that women who are taking HRT orally have a two-four times increased risk of developing a blood clot than those not taking HRT

- The overall risk of HRT oral users developing blood clots is normally very low

- studies have estimated that for every 1,000 women using oral HRT tablets for 7.5 years, just less than two will develop a blood clot

Heart Disease and Strokes

According to NICE:

- the use of HRT does not increase the risk of developing cardiovascular disease (including heart disease and strokes) if started before the age 60.

- HRT which is oestrogen-only has no, or reduced risk of heart disease

- HRT which is combined has little or no increased risk of heart disease

- a small increased risk of stroke is linked to taking HRT oestrogen-only tablets, the normal risk for women that have a stroke under the age of 60 is very low therefore the risk is small

If you are considering taking HRT do make an appointment to discuss it in depth with your GP. They will perform a full health check and discuss any of your concerns regarding the risks associated with the use of HRT.

Types of HRT available:

- tablet form taken orally - daily
- a patch to be applied to the skin. These are very popular, they deliver a constant absorption of hormone through the skin, they are more preferred as they are not absorbed through the liver therefore reducing the risk of blood clots.
- HRT gel – simply applied to the skin
- Mirena coil – the coil contains a form of progesterone. The coil is inserted into the womb.
- Pessaries – Oestrogen can be taken in the form of a pessary which is inserted into the vagina. A vaginal ring can also be inserted into the vagina as another alternative to receive HRT.
- Local oestrogen therapy – This can be in the form of a vaginal tablet called Vagifem, or a cream such as Gynest or Ovestin. These are known to help with symptoms such as painful sex and vaginal dryness. These are used by ladies who can't or don't wish to use the systemic HRT. These are very low dose therapies so equivalent of having one HRT tablet every six months

Testosterone Treatment for Menopause

On occasion, doctors do additionally prescribe the male hormone testosterone if there are no benefits from using the oestrogen replacement. Testosterone can improve energy levels and libido. Your GP will give you more information.

Bioidentical Hormones - Due to the cancer scares linked to synthetic HRT the interest of a more natural HRT has now steered towards bioidentical hormone therapy. These bioidentical hormones are said to be identical in molecular structure to the natural hormones made in the woman's own body. Bioidentical hormones are synthesized from a plant chemical taken from yams and soy. The bioidentical oestrogens are 17 beta-estradiol, estriol and estrone. Estradiol is the form of oestrogen which depletes during menopause. Bioidentical progesterone is finely ground in the laboratory to aid in better absorption in the body.

QUESTION – "Are bioidentical hormones or natural hormones safer than the traditional HRT used for menopausal symptoms?" "Are they more effective?"

According to the Food and Drug Administration (FDA) and various other medical specialty groups the answer is – "No, they are not!" They go on to say that the hormones advertised as "bioidentical" and "natural" are not safer than the traditional HRT normally used. There is no evidence that they are more effective.

"Bioidentical" is stating that the hormones within the product are chemically identical to the hormones produced in the body. The hormones in the bioidentical therapy medications may not be any different to those in the traditional HRT.

The word "natural" means that the hormones in the product are derived from animal or plant sources; they are not created or synthesized in a laboratory. These so called "natural" products are being commercially processed to become bioidentical.

Traditional HRT do not exclude natural hormones. FDA-approved products such as – Vivelle-Dot, Climera and Estrace that contain oestrogens and Prometrium – a natural progesterone - are also derived from plants.

The creators of bioidentical hormones state their products have advantages over traditional HRT:

- **Our bioidentical hormones are produced in forms and doses that are different from the ones approved by the FDA.** One would need to go through a compounding pharmacy to acquire these products. This pharmacy would specialize in tailoring these medications to suit the woman's individual needs. The problem is that these products from compounding pharmacies haven't been tested to the same rigorous quality assurance standards that commercially available hormonal treatments must meet to be approved.
- **Bioidentical hormones are tailor made especially to the individual. This is based on a saliva test to assess one's unique hormonal levels.** However, the hormone levels in the saliva do not reflect the levels of hormones found in the blood or correspond to the menopause symptoms.

As you can see there are very muddy waters here but is any medication really 100% safe? If it is FDA-APPROVED we have a kind of peace of mind but any medication we take is taken at our own risk regardless of just how approved it may be. The body loves natural and not synthetic in any form.

There are many women who are benefiting from customized doses and forms of bioidentical hormone products but it still stands that there is no scientific support of these compounds over commercially produced preparations. There are women who have tried the bioidentical route and have had awful side effects.

The benefits of taking the traditional HRT for the vast majority of women under 60 years of age do outweigh the risks. For younger women who have experienced an early menopause HRT is recommended to them which they can take until they are at least 51 years of age. The length of time to be using HRT really depends on the woman herself, the doctor will guide their patient and monitor their health regularly. It could take a couple or few tries of using various HRT methods as 'one kind will not suit all'. Taking HRT early when needed really can make a positive difference to the symptoms and quality of life. It will also contribute to protecting bone and heart health.

HRT and Hysterectomy

A total hysterectomy means the surgical removal of the whole of the womb (or uterus) and the cervix. A sub-total hysterectomy is the removal of the uterus only leaving the cervix intact. A hysterectomy with bi-lateral salpingo oophorectomy means the removal of the womb, ovaries and fallopian tubes.

Women who have had a hysterectomy would usually need oestrogen and possibly testosterone therapy. When a woman has had a hysterectomy plus oophorectomy (removal of ovaries) this means that the oestrogen production (originally from her ovaries) will cease although small amounts of oestrogen will still be produced from the adrenal glands and fatty tissues. The menopause will now begin and oestrogen deficiency must be avoided by treatment to avoid further health issues.

If a hysterectomy is performed that leaves the ovaries in place there is a 50% chance of ovarian failure within 5 years of the operation. One of the major issues of undergoing a surgical menopause (hysterectomy) is to decide if you wish to take Hormone Replacement Therapy. HRT can be very helpful in alleviating the many symptoms of menopause. It is also important for a woman to understand that her body is now without the natural protection of the female sex hormones and will now have an increased risk of Alzheimer's disease, heart disease and osteoporosis.

Factors in favour of taking HRT include:
- severe climacteric symptom
- family history of heart disease
- high risk category related to heart disease
- family history of osteoporosis
- high risk category of osteoporosis

The HRT given to women who have had a hysterectomy is oestrogen-only although it is possible to be given treatment to replace testosterone too. When starting HRT for the first time, it is normal to be prescribed the lowest dose which will then be increased if necessary to fully alleviate menopausal symptoms. This still may not give enough oestrogen to protect a woman's heart and bone health. Women who have had hysterectomies before the age of 40 will require more oestrogen as their bodies were producing more before the operation.

Women do decide against taking HRT for the following reasons:

- high risk category of thrombosis
- family history of thrombosis
- history of thrombosis
- high risk category related to breast cancer
- family history of breast cancer
- history of breast cancer

Chapter 8.

A Natural Approach to Managing the Menopause

****Always consult a healthcare professional before taking any form of herbal remedies or supplements. Here are some guidelines but this is not intended to replace medical advice:**

- If you have a health problem always consult your doctor for a diagnosis, always check with your doctor before starting any herbal supplements as they can interact with medications
- Do not use herbal remedies when pregnant or breastfeeding unless under the supervision of a medical professional
- Herbal remedies must not be used by children under 2 years of age unless under the supervision of a medical professional
- Never exceed the recommended doses
- Do not take if taking medication – always speak to your doctor first
- Do not take more than 3 herbal remedies concurrently
- Always stop taking herbal remedies at least 21 days before surgery

More and more women are now turning to self-help approaches to managing their menopause journey. Here are some natural alternatives:

Herbs – Sage is a very useful remedy when needing relief from hot flushes and night sweats. This herb is well known for its culinary uses but is also thought to be beneficial in re-balancing the sweat-regulating mechanism in the brain bringing the temperature back to normal.

The medicinal history of sage goes back eons, the Romans believed it to be sacred and the Chinese would trade tea in exchange for supplies of sage of which they used medicinally.
Recent research has shown that taking sage extracts can help to reduce anxiety, increase mental performance, promote calmness and a feeling of great well-being. sage doesn't affect the hormones in any way so is safe to use with HRT however ladies are using it without HRT alongside other natural treatments. If you have sage growing in your herb garden then you can make your own tea, add a little manuka honey to sweeten. The health food stores sell the pre-made sage tea bags too.

SOY - is a natural source of estrogen. Soy has been well studied for its effect on relieving muscle pain as well as vaginal dryness. Research has suggested that adding soy to the diet can be almost effective as taking HRT.

GMO Soy – Since 1994 there has been an increasing volume of foods being developed using genetic modification (GMO). GMO has sparked much controversy, especially in Europe where the concern is high regarding the safety of consuming GMO foods. Approximately half of the american soybean crop which was planted in 1999 carried a gene that makes it resistant to a herbicide (Roundup) used to control weeds.

Dong Quai – is highly recommended to be used to balance oestrogen levels. It can re-balance oestrogen levels as they fluctuate. Dong Quai has been used for centuries in traditional Chinese medicine as a treatment for the health of female hormones and to ease PMS symptoms. Studies have shown that dong quai contains compounds that can support and treat menopausal symptoms. Dong quai is available in health food stores in the form of a capsule, tablet or liquid.

Hawthorne – A common complaint of many women going through the menopause are low blood pressure and an irregular heartbeat.
Always see your doctor to have your condition checked thoroughly and confirmed. If your problems are due to the menopause then hawthorne can help. Hawthorne is a plant which has anti-arrhythmic compounds which will help to control your heartbeat. This amazing plant can dilate the arteries which provides blood flow to the heart. This can help to reduce the risk of heart attack and can also reduce the very uncomfortable feeling of palpitations. If the blood pressure is too low, hawthorne can help to stabilize this too.

Black Cohosh – is a herb that is classed as the gold standard in alleviating menopausal symptoms naturally. The Native American tribes use this herb as a medicine for painful periods, in labour and childbirth and menopause symptoms.

Many women all around the world use Black Cohosh especially for night sweats and hot flushes. It also said to help with depression and vaginal dryness. Black Cohosh is the highest recommended herb as an alternative remedy to HRT. Research has shown an improvement in menopausal symptoms in 80% of women using black cohosh within six to eight weeks.

Alfalfa – is a herb which is very rich in minerals and nutrients. Women have reported that their use of this herb has helped with their menopausal symptoms, especially with mood swings although there are very few scientific studies to support these reports. This herb is reported to be a balancing herb as it can boost low oestrogen levels and reduce high oestrogen levels. It can also aid in reducing the blood cholesterol to a healthy level. The body loves natural.

Evening Primrose – is a highly affective herb and has been used since the 1930s. It is used as a treatment for inflammatory conditions, skin conditions, diabetes and even in deterring certain cancers. The oils from the plant seeds are used to relieve night sweats, PMS, mood swings and breast pain. Studies have proved that evening primrose as a supplement can be very effective against menopause symptoms such as hot flushes and headaches.

Valerian Root – like many other herbs has been used for hundreds of years for many different reasons. This herb has been used for insomnia, migraines, headaches, convulsions and body aches. Valerian root relieves hot flushes, muscle tension, anxiety attacks and hot flushes.

Chasteberry – is packed with antioxidant properties to help to remove free radicals in the body. It also has an anti-inflammatory effect. It used for digestive disorders as well as reducing blood cholesterol levels. There are studies which have shown that the use of chasteberry extract could help with pre-menopausal symptoms and at the early stage of menopause. Chasteberry contains hormone balancing properties.

Red Clover – is a herbal remedy used to ease menopausal hot flushes and night sweats. It is also known as cow clover, meadow clover and wild clover.
There are weak oestrogen substances found in red clover and these are known as daidzein, genistein, formononetin and biochanin. These plant hormones are similar to the phytoestrogens found in soy. Women who live in Asia usually have a diet rich in soy and it is found that they report less menopausal symptoms than women in the west.

Ginseng – is a herb which is adaptogenic and this is a natural substance that supports the body to adapt to stress. It also contains saponins and ginsenosides which are antioxidant and anti-inflammatory properties. Ginseng has the ability to increase the neurotransmitters – dopamine and serotonin in the brain, these are known as the feel-good chemicals. This effect improves the mood and the ability to fight off insomnia. Research states that ginseng may have similar properties to oestrogen. Small quantities of estrone, estradiol and estriol are found in the ginseng root. Balanced oestrogen levels can help to reduce insomnia and mood swings experience by menopausal women.

Milk Thistle – is a cleansing herb which is used by many women going through the menopause. The active ingredient in milk thistle is a bioflavonoid called silymarin, this can help to support hormonal balance because of its protective action on the liver. Milk thistle can also protect against some female cancers.

Ginko Biloba – is used by many women looking for a natural alternative remedy rather than HRT. Numerous studies have shown that the standardized ginko extract does possess oestrogen activity and may be an appropriate substitute for HRT. Ginko biloba can help menopausal women in various ways such as improving blood flow to the brain and other major organs. This can be a huge benefit as low levels of oestrogen do contribute to problems such as poor memory performance and forgetfulness.

The benefits of ginko biloba are:
- nourishing brain cells
- boosting oxygen levels in the brain
- supporting cognitive function
- improving concentration

- supporting and improving memory capacity

Essential Foods and Vitamins

Vitamin D – It is important to understand that although women are being prescribed HRT as a preventative treatment against developing osteoporosis, supporting bone density does not rely on a perfect balance of hormones alone. There are essential nutrients needed too and vitamin D is one of them. Calcium is needed daily for bone health. Calcium absorption depends on vitamin D and this is made through our skin activated by sunlight. As we age, our ability to absorb vitamin D decreases plus the food sources are limited. It is very important to take a daily supplement and it is recommended to take 1000-2000 iu per day of the D3 form. Check this with your doctor first.

Vitamin E – Approximately 75% of menopausal women suffer from hot flushes. Research has shown that by taking 400IU of vitamin E per day, there has been a significant reduction in the severity and frequency of hot flush attacks. This daily supplement has also shown a positive effect on reducing vaginal dryness. If you decide to take a supplement form then do buy one which contains d-alpha-tocopherol as this is easily absorbed.

B Vitamins – can help to support your nervous system, especially if you are suffering from depression, anxiety, panic attacks and stress. B vitamins are known as the 'stress nutrients' and help to produce the feel-good neurotransmitter serotonin.

They also help the adrenal glands to adapt to and manage stress. B vitamins work in harmony together so it is best to choose a B complex supplement which provides all the essential B vitamins such as B1 to B6, B12 and folic acid. Foods rich in B vitamins include meat, fish, eggs, green leafy vegetables, dairy and fortified foods.

Omega 3 essential fatty acids – are essential to help support the hormone balance and they have a lubricating effect on the body. The signs of omega 3 deficiency are similar to the symptoms experienced during the menopause such as, aching joints, depression, fatigue and dry skin. Omega 3 have also been linked to lowering the risk of breast cancer. Omega 3 rich foods include green leafy vegetables, seeds, nuts and oily fish (fresh tuna, seafood, sardines, herring, mackerel and salmon).

Phytoestrogenic Foods – may help to alleviate symptoms of menopause due to their effect on oestrogen receptors at the cell membrane. When oestrogen levels are low, they attach to the receptors and stimulate a mild oestroegenic action. If there is an excess of oestrogen, the phytoestrogens block the cell receptors. Foods rich in phytoestrogens are, celery, parsley, fennel, garlic, mungbeans, linseeds, lentils and soya (miso, tofu and tempeh).

Chapter 9.

The positives of Post-Menopause living

Post-menopause life can be as healthy as we wish it to be. A strong support system is essential for optimal spiritual growth. Friendships, family relationships and loving oneself is very important to grow with great health and a strong mindset. Love is the most powerful force of nature and to love and be loved is ever so important now. Post-menopause marks the end of the menstrual cycle which for the vast majority of women is a huge blessing. Post-menopause can be very liberating especially for those women who have been plagued with heavy bleeding which has been irregular and painful. This eliminates the hassle of using tampons or pads, no more being tied to the house to be near to the toilet – "just in case." No more premenstrual syndrome (PMS)! PMS can be debilitating and very isolating for the sufferer. This condition will not be missed. Post-menopause women can have intercourse with peace of mind that they can no longer get pregnant. Women have reported the best sex life ever at this stage of their lives.

Say goodbye to the hormonal headaches which have plagued women throughout their menopausal journey. Women are affected by migraines three times more than men according to the National Headache Foundation. Approximately 70% of these women suffer from menstrual migraines and headaches that coincide with ovulation and menstruation. These headaches can be accompanied by nausea, vomiting and light/sound sensitivity. Once the hormones stop fluctuating as in the menopause, the headaches and migraines do decrease but once in the post-menopause stage these issues will (hopefully) be no more.

It is very common for women to develop fibroids as they approach their 50s. Fibroids are uterine tumours which are usually almost benign. Thankfully, once women reach menopause/post-menopause these fibroids often shrink and stop growing as the oestrogen levels decline.

Post-menopausal women experience what they call the **"menopausal zest"** – which is described as a renewal or refreshing of all areas of their lives. It is a time to reflect on how happy they feel with whom they have become and accepting the changes that must be made to enable their dreams and ambitions to come to fruition. They say they feel a rush of newfound energy both mentally and physically which can take them on a more meaningful chapter in their lives.

Many women decide to take a fresh look at the relationships in their lives, their professions and how they are nurturing themselves. Women also report that they become more self-analyzing and begin to question each are of their lives as in "do my relationships serve me well?" "Am I happy and fulfilled in my career?" "Is it time to take my life in a new direction?" Post-menopause can be a very liberating and empowering stage in a woman's life if approached with care and with self-belief.

It can either be a mid-life crisis or a mid-life chrysalis emerging into a more healthy, self-confident and inspiring individual – we all have a choice in which road to travel down – choose it wisely.

To think that we have another 40-50 years of life left to live in our post-menopause years is one very enriching thought. We have masses of experience and wisdom which we can now use to build a richer existence. The body can be created into a new, healthy and beautiful image and relationships can take on a whole new meaning for us. Life will be valued in a more meaningful way. Our health and diet will be our top priority especially now our children are grown and time is (hopefully) coming back to us. Regular exercise, pampering, nurturing, loving and living.

There will always be women who will find the menopause journey very difficult, it can overwhelm them and make them feel very alone and isolated – if allowed. There are countless women out there in the world who will have the role of "carer" for their loved ones and may not have a strong support system. Again, one must look for help and support, it is usually out there somewhere, having a positive attitude and learning to take care of "you" counts more than ever before. There will always be life stresses, the healthier we are in body and mind, the less we will struggle.

Thinking Positively

I often think about the awesome surgeons, doctors and nurses working long shifts in a pressured and emotional environment. They too will have their own life tragedies and general daily life stressors to deal with but they do continue day after day working tirelessly to serve and care for hundreds of thousands of people in need. We just need to think for a little while each day, appreciate and respect the lives of others and their contributions. Every day look at your glass being half full and not half empty, count your blessings each morning before you begin your day. Regret, anger and frustration will break down the spirit resulting in illness and disease.

When I am stuck in the traffic jam, I can feel my impatience creeping in so I remind myself to STOP and steer my mind back to the presence of being thankful to all of you out there! I am then released from a negative and have entered a new positive. Parents, family and close friends are our best source of comfort but if this support is too limited then it is important to take big action and look for ways to start to build yourself healthy new relationships/friendships. Join a women's group or sign up at your nearest College to take on a new course for a fresh challenge. Friendship is most important especially now when life is giving you a challenging menopause map to navigate through

A course of cognitive behavioural therapy is very useful as it can re-wire our thought processes from feelings of hopelessness to a newfound feeling of liberation and spiritual freedom. There are many self-help books which are great tools to use whilst dealing with uncomfortable feelings and issues. Take on a new hobby that you have set aside over the years, make it a priority. Meeting new people is stimulating and helps to grow self-confidence. Be pro-active in your self-growth, you are your very best friend. Think of this stage in your life as a reinvention of your mind, body and soul.

I have always raised my sons to never judge people by how they look, so why should we be judged because of our age? So many of us are fighting against the natural process of ageing but why not take a different approach? Think of ageing as a gift in that there is no more pressure to have to exert our efforts and purse-strings just to look an ideal or expected way to be more acceptable to others.

I often think back to my 20s and the amount of money I would spend on make-up and fashion just to look like the models out of the magazines. Did it make me happy? It certainly did not. Did it make me healthy? It certainly did not as I was usually suffering from the after-effects of late nights, the effects of alcohol, the effects of eating the wrong foods not to mention an empty bank account. I would certainly do things very different if I could go back, but wouldn't we all? We now have this pressure removed, we can now be the healthiest and most fulfilled we have ever been and for the right reasons. This thought helped me hugely and this helped me to accept my face and body ageing with grace, I feel liberated for the first time in my life so a big thank-you to the ageing process (chink chink).

It is still a fact that saying goodbye to the first part of our life can be sad at times as I am sure there are women out there who miss their youthful face and body, many do complain on how the natural ageing process makes us feel less feminine and how it can negatively affect our self-esteem. I was one of those women, but my mindset was the first thing I had to re-programme. I knew I had to now practice a tougher discipline with my food choices, cutting out alcohol, my exercise routine and my overall lifestyle.

I started to read more self-help books on self-esteem, self-confidence, eliminating stress from my life and personal transformation. I sought a councilor to help with my acceptance of new health challenges and ageing, I grieved in a safe place but oh boy did it help. I felt like I had found a whole new me. So, we must take whatever measures necessary to put value on our life and to be healthy for ourselves and our loved ones. Don't sweat the small stuff as after-all... it is usually small stuff. Laugh at life and life will be so much more enjoyable for you. Count your blessings, look around you and be thankful for all you have. Always see the glass as half full – not half empty. Negative thoughts materialize into a negative life so practice positive thinking always. Life is a gift and we must cherish it – while we have it.

Conclusion

I do hope you enjoyed my book, it is the first book I have written and I have had many sleepless nights over it. I have tried to cover as much of the menopause topic as I possibly could without it being too long a read.

Please may I ask if you would be so kind as to leave an honest review on behalf of this book on Amazon as this will help me to become a more established author. The more positive reviews the book has, the more visible it will be to other readers.

If the reviews are somewhat negative I will certainly do whatever it takes to improve the information required. I would greatly appreciate your honesty and feedback. Thank-you sincerely.